STRETCHING EXERCISES FOR SENIORS OVER 60

2024/2025

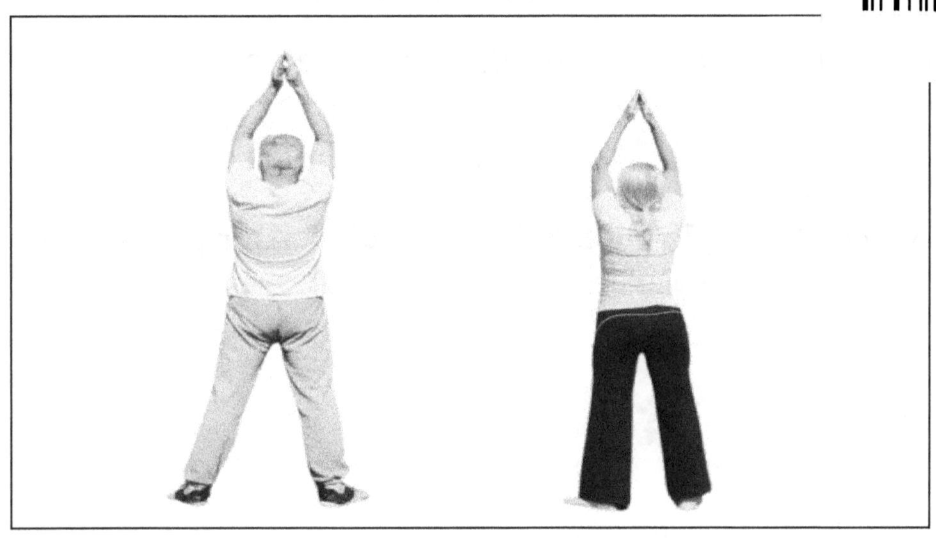

Quick Guide Workout to boost mobility, vitality and enhance balance to prevent injuries during Aging days

Lyndon S. Vergara

COPYRIGHT

Before this document is duplicated or reproduced in any manner, the publisher's consent must be gained. Therefore, the contents within can neither be stored electronically, transferred, nor kept in a database. Neither in Part nor full can the document be copied, scanned, faxed, or retained without approval from the publisher or creator.

TABLE OF CONTENTS

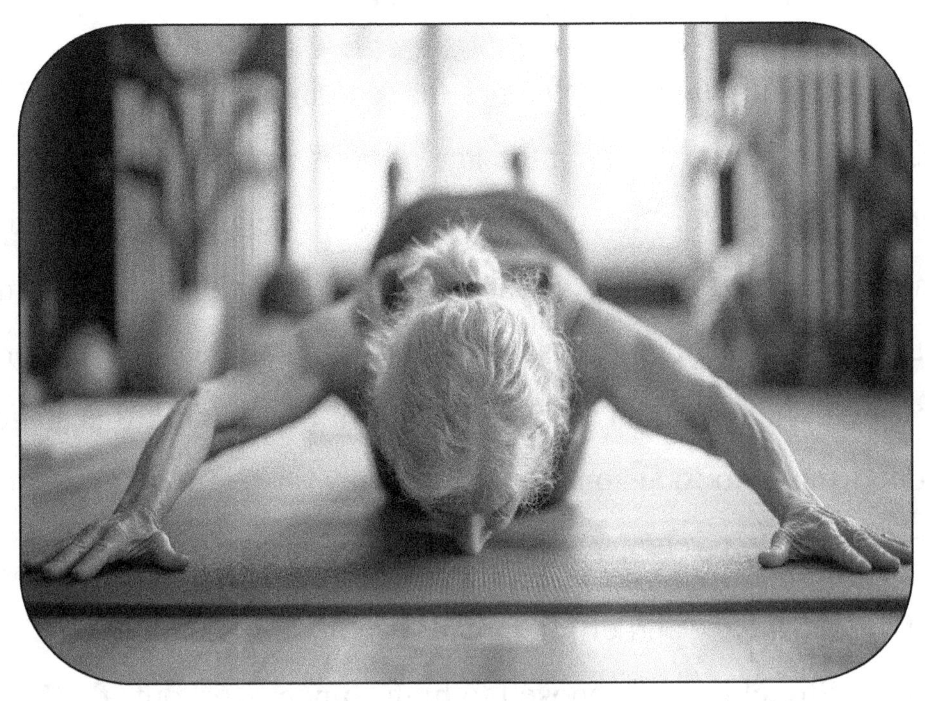

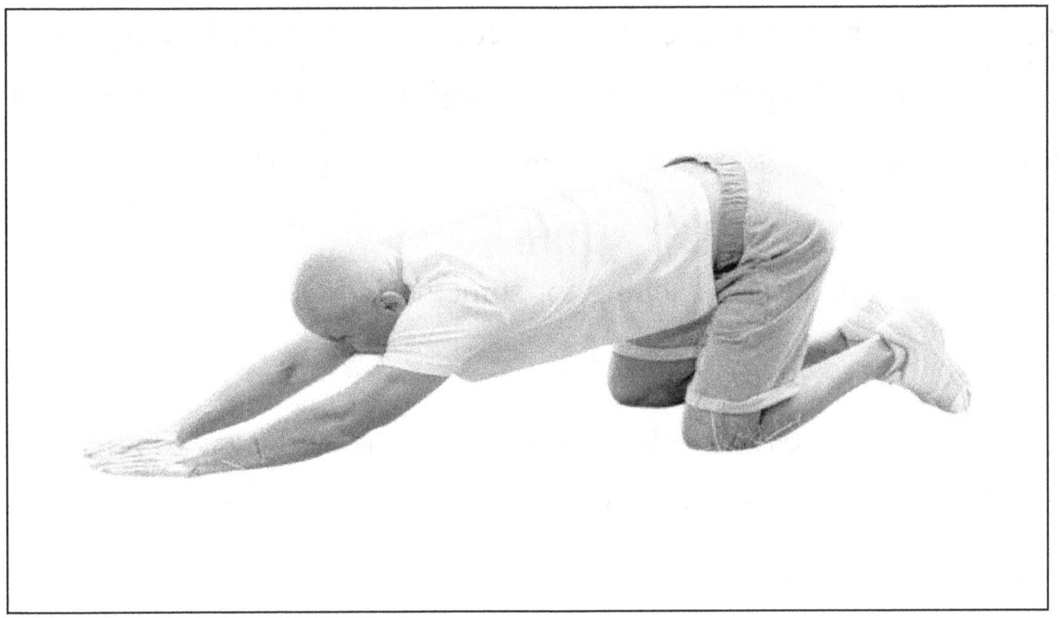

INTRODUCTION

As we age, our bodies naturally undergo changes that can impact our mobility, balance, and overall well-being. For many, reaching the age of 60 is a milestone that comes with a mix of pride and concern, pride for the years lived and experiences gained, and concern for the physical limitations that often accompany aging. While it's true that aging can bring challenges such as joint stiffness, muscle weakness, and a decrease in bone density, it doesn't have to mean giving up on an active and vibrant life. In fact, this stage of life presents a unique opportunity to focus on our health and well-being in ways we might have overlooked in our younger years.

Stretching is one of the most easy and efficient ways to prevent the physical consequences of aging. Stretching, as opposed to high-impact workouts that can put strain on aging joints and bones, is a low-impact activity that can be tailored to your specific requirements and capabilities. Regular stretching helps to maintain and even develop flexibility, which is necessary for performing daily tasks with ease and confidence. Flexibility is essential for moving freely and comfortably, whether you're bending down to tie your shoes, reaching for something on a high shelf, or getting up from a chair.

Stretching not only improves flexibility but also promotes muscle and joint health. As we age, our muscles gradually lose strength and suppleness, increasing our susceptibility to accidents and falls. Stretching helps to prevent this by increasing muscle tone and range of motion, decreasing stiffness, and promoting proper posture and alignment. It also increases circulation, which is necessary for supplying oxygen and nutrients to your muscles and joints, aiding in recuperation and sustaining function. People over the age of 60 are at a higher risk of having illnesses including arthritis and osteoporosis. These diseases can cause discomfort, limited movement, and an increased risk of fractures and other injuries. Regular stretching can help to reduce these risks by keeping joints flexible and minimizing inflammation. Stretching activities, particularly those that involve light weight-bearing, can help improve bone health by increasing density and strength. This is especially crucial in reducing falls and fractures, which are common and often crippling injuries among elderly.

This book is designed to be a thorough guide to preserving and enhancing your flexibility, balance, and total mobility after 60. Each chapter will give you realistic, easy-to-follow stretching regimens targeted to the specific needs of seniors. You'll learn how to do each stretch safely and effectively, including adaptations for people with unique limits or ailments. You'll also get advice on how to incorporate these routines into your daily life, making stretching a fun and sustainable aspect of your journey to greater health.

CHAPTER 1: THE IMPORTANCE OF STAYING FLEXIBLE AFTER 60

Why Stretching Matters

One of the most important advantages of stretching for seniors is its capacity to maintain and enhance flexibility. Stretching keeps muscles supple as they age, minimizing stiffness and discomfort in daily movements. This increased flexibility is required for everyday actions like reaching for objects, bending over, and rising from a seated position, all of which can become more difficult with age. Stretching also helps to prevent injuries, which is especially important for elders. As joints and muscles weaken, the risk of strains, sprains, and other injuries rises. Regular stretching helps to preserve the range of motion in joints and muscles, making them less vulnerable to injury. Stretching also improves blood circulation, which helps deliver critical nutrients to muscles and joints, resulting in faster recovery and better overall health.

Stretching can also improve balance. A loss of balance in seniors can lead to falls, which are the main cause of injury in this demographic. Stretching exercises, particularly those aimed at strengthening core and lower body muscles, can improve stability and coordination, lowering the risk of falling. Furthermore, stretching provides psychological and emotional benefits. Regular stretching habits promote mindfulness and relaxation, which can help reduce stress and anxiety, two prevalent difficulties among seniors. Stretching is a vital activity for seniors who want to live active, satisfying lives far into their golden years since it promotes physical health and a sense of wellbeing.

Benefits of Stretching for Seniors

1. Improved Flexibility and Range of Motion

As our bodies age, our muscles and joints naturally lose flexibility, which can make regular tasks more difficult. Stretching on a regular basis helps to maintain and enhance flexibility, making it simpler to execute everyday movements like bending, reaching, and twisting. This increased range of motion improves general mobility while lowering the risk of muscle strains and joint problems.

2. Enhanced Balance and Stability

Stretching helps enhance balance and stability by strengthening the muscles surrounding the joints, particularly in the legs and core. This is critical for seniors since balance tends to deteriorate with age, increasing the risk of falls, the largest cause of injury among older persons. Stretching exercises that emphasize balance and coordination can help seniors keep their independence and confidence in their movements.

3. Reduced Pain and Stiffness

Stretching relieves muscular and joint stiffness, a prevalent problem among elderly. Stretching can help relieve pain from illnesses including arthritis, back pain, and general muscle tightness by extending tight muscles and releasing tension. Stretching on a regular basis improves circulation to the muscles and joints, reducing inflammation and promoting recovery.

4. Improved Circulation

Stretching improves blood flow throughout the body, bringing more oxygen and nutrients to the muscles and tissues. This enhanced circulation can help with healing, relieve muscle tightness, and improve general physical health. Better circulation also helps to prevent problems like deep vein thrombosis, which can be problematic for less active seniors.

5. Increased Muscle Strength and Endurance

Stretching generally increases flexibility, but it also boosts muscle strength and endurance, especially when combined with resistance workouts. Stronger muscles support and protect joints, minimizing stress on them during regular activities. This can result in enhanced functional fitness, helping elders to stay active and complete chores more readily.

6. Mental and Emotional Benefits

Stretching benefits both the body and the mind. It promotes relaxation and awareness, reducing tension, anxiety, and sadness. Stretching habitual nature can create a sense of calm and control, resulting in improved mental health and emotional well-being.

7. Prevention of Injuries

Regular stretching prepares the body for exercise by warming up muscles and boosting flexibility, lowering the risk of injury. Stretching before and after physical exercises can help prevent strains, sprains, and muscle tears, so it's an essential part of any senior fitness plan.

8. Support for Overall Health and Well-being

Stretching assists seniors in being active, which is critical for general health and lifespan. Staying physically active can help seniors manage chronic disorders like diabetes, heart disease, and osteoporosis, as well as improve their quality of life by allowing them to participate in their favorite activities with more ease and comfort.

Overcoming Common Misconceptions About Aging and Flexibility

Misconception 1: "It's Normal to Lose Flexibility and There's Nothing You Can Do About It"

One of the most common misconceptions is that losing flexibility is a natural aspect of aging and that nothing can be done to avoid it. While some normal changes occur in muscles and joints as we age, such as decreasing muscle mass and joint stiffness, these changes do not indicate a complete loss of flexibility. Flexibility can deteriorate if not actively maintained; however, including regular stretching and mobility exercises into a daily routine will help preserve and even enhance flexibility. The body adapts throughout life, and with constant effort, seniors can retain or recover a wide range of mobility.

Misconception 2: "Stretching is Only for Athletes or Younger People"

Many seniors feel that stretching is only for sports or young people who are physically active. This is a serious misconception. Stretching is good for everyone, no matter their age or fitness level. Stretching might be especially important for seniors since it helps prevent the natural age-related reductions in muscle flexibility and joint mobility. Gentle stretching targeted to the needs of older persons can increase flexibility, lower the risk of injury, and improve overall quality of life.

Misconception 3: "Stretching is Too Difficult or Painful for Older Adults"

Another prevalent myth is that stretching is excessively difficult or uncomfortable for the elderly. While some stretching exercises might be difficult, particularly for individuals with limited mobility or chronic diseases, there are numerous mild stretches intended expressly for older adults that are both safe and beneficial. To avoid overexertion, focus on good technique and heed to your body's cues. Stretching should never produce discomfort; if it does, it may be because the stretch is being performed incorrectly or is too advanced for the individual's current capacity. Beginning with basic stretches and progressively progressing will help increase confidence and flexibility while minimizing discomfort.

Misconception 4: "You Can't Improve Flexibility After a Certain Age"

Many people assume that once flexibility is lost, it cannot be recovered, especially in later life. However, this is not correct. While aging reduces the body's flexibility, it is never too late to begin stretching and enhancing your range of motion. According to research, older persons who engage in regular stretching and flexibility training have considerable increases in their flexibility, strength, and overall mobility. The body is extremely adaptive, and with persistent, conscious practice, flexibility may be increased at any age.

Misconception 5: "Stretching Alone Won't Make a Difference"

Some seniors may believe that stretching alone will not have a substantial impact on their overall fitness or health. Stretching, on the other hand, is an essential action that underpins all other types of movement and exercise. Stretching improves flexibility, making it simpler to do daily tasks, engage in physical activity, and lower the chance of injury. Stretching also improves circulation, relieves muscle tension, and promotes relaxation, which benefits both physical and mental health.

Misconception 6: "You Need Special Equipment or a Gym Membership to Stretch Effectively"

There is a misperception that successful stretching necessitates special equipment or access to a gym. In actuality, stretching is one of the most accessible kinds of exercise because it takes little or no equipment. Many excellent stretches can be done at home on a chair, a wall, or the floor. A yoga mat or resistance bands can provide some support, but they are not required. The most crucial part of stretching is consistency and appropriate technique, rather than flashy equipment.

Misconception 7: "Stretching is a Waste of Time"

Finally, some seniors may see stretching as a waste of time, especially if they don't see instant results. Stretching can provide more subtle and cumulative advantages than more rigorous forms of exercise. However, frequent stretching has major long-term benefits, including increased flexibility, decreased discomfort, improved posture, and enhanced balance. These benefits can significantly improve a senior's ability to keep active, avoid accidents, and maintain independence.

CHAPTER 2: UNDERSTANDING YOUR BODY'S CHANGING NEEDS

How Aging Affects Your Muscles and Joints

Our bodies naturally change as we age, which can have an influence on our muscles and joints. Understanding these changes is critical for people over the age of 60 who want to manage and improve their physical health. Here's an in-depth look at how aging affects muscles and joints, as well as what you can do to address the changes.

1. Decreased Muscle Mass and Strength

One of the most visible impacts of aging on the muscles is the steady decrease of muscular mass, often known as sarcopenia. Muscle mass normally begins to drop around the age of 30, and this process accelerates as we age. By the time people reach their 60s and beyond, this loss of muscle mass can become more noticeable. This drop is the result of a number of reasons, including decreased physical activity, hormonal changes, and changes in muscle protein synthesis. Muscle strength diminishes with muscle mass, affecting your capacity to execute daily activities and maintain balance.

What You Can Do: Regular resistance training and strength workouts can help prevent muscle loss. Activities like bodyweight exercises, resistance bands, or modest weights can help enhance muscle strength and function. Even modest strength exercise can be quite effective at preserving muscle mass and improving general mobility.

2. Reduced Muscle Elasticity

Muscle fibers become less elastic and flexible as we age. This loss in suppleness can cause muscles to feel stiffer and more vulnerable to injury. Reduced elasticity is generally caused by changes in the connective tissues within the muscles, such as decreased collagen formation. This rigidity can limit range of motion and increase the risk of strains and sprains.

What You Can Do: Muscle elasticity can be maintained and improved with regular stretching and flexibility exercises. Stretching techniques can help prevent stiffness and promote a wider range of motion. Gentle yoga and stretching activities can be very effective at improving muscle flexibility and reducing tension.

3. Joint Degeneration and Stiffness

Another prevalent aging-related concern is joint deterioration. Cartilage, the smooth tissue that cushions the joints, can wear away over time, resulting in disorders like osteoarthritis. This deterioration causes more friction between bones, resulting in pain, stiffness, and restricted joint motion. Furthermore, the synovial fluid that lubricates the joints may diminish, resulting in increased discomfort and stiffness.

What You Can Do: Low-impact workouts like swimming, cycling, and walking can assist maintain joint health without putting too much strain on the joints. Stretching activities aimed at increasing joint mobility can also be beneficial. Resistance exercise can help to strengthen the muscles around the joints and lessen strain on them.

4. Decreased Bone Density

Aging also has an impact on bone density, with many older persons losing bone mass, a condition known as osteoporosis. Bone density declines, making bones more weak and prone to fracture. Hormonal changes, a lack of physical exercise, and an insufficient intake of important minerals such as calcium and vitamin D all contribute to a decrease in bone density.

What You Can Do: Weight-bearing workouts like walking, dancing, and resistance training can help you maintain your bone density and strength. Furthermore, ensuring an appropriate amount of calcium and vitamin D through food or supplementation might benefit bone health. It is also recommended that you consult with a healthcare specialist to receive tailored bone health suggestions.

5. Slower Recovery and Healing

Aging also reduces the body's ability to heal from traumas and repair damaged tissues. Reduced blood supply, less cell regeneration, and slower metabolic processes all contribute to the sluggish recovery. This means that healing durations from accidents or muscular strains may be greater in older persons than in younger people.

What You Can Do: Prioritizing healthy nutrition, water, and adequate rest can help the body repair. Gentle workouts and stretching can improve circulation and help with healing. Furthermore, being cognizant of progressive progression in physical activity can minimize overexertion and lower the chance of injury.

The Role of Flexibility in Mobility and Balance

1. Enhanced Range of Motion

Flexibility refers to the ability of muscles and joints to move across their whole range of motion. Maintaining flexibility in seniors helps to keep their muscles and joints nimble and capable of executing routine activities. This increased range of motion is required for actions like reaching, bending, twisting, and climbing stairs. Without proper flexibility, these basic actions can become more difficult, resulting in decreased independence.

Example: Seniors' shoulder and hip flexibility allows them to reach for objects on high shelves or elevate their legs over obstacles more easily, lowering the risk of strains and enhancing overall functionality.

2. Improved Posture and Alignment

Good flexibility helps to maintain correct posture and body alignment. As we age, muscular imbalances and stiffness can cause poor posture, which can be uncomfortable and contribute to back and neck pain. Stretching and flexibility exercises help to properly align the body by extending tight muscles and strengthening weak ones. Improved posture not only relieves discomfort but also improves balance by distributing the body's weight evenly.

Example: Stretching the chest and upper back helps alleviate the consequences of extended sitting and bad posture, resulting in a more upright and balanced stance.

3. Better Balance and Stability

Flexibility has a direct impact on balance and stability. Tight muscles and tight joints might impair the capacity to quickly react to changes in posture or movement, increasing the risk of falling. Flexible muscles and joints enable smoother, more controlled movements, which are critical for maintaining balance. Stretching exercises for the legs, hips, and core can help strengthen the muscles responsible for stability and improve overall balance.

Example: Increased ankle and leg flexibility can help seniors keep their balance when walking on uneven ground or making rapid movements, lowering the chance of falling.

4. Prevention of Injuries

Flexibility helps to prevent injuries by allowing the body to move freely and lowering the danger of overstretching or straining muscles and joints. Flexibility exercises can provide protection for seniors who already have reduced muscular strength or joint health. Seniors can avoid unnecessary stress and strain during daily activities by keeping their muscles and joints supple.

Example: Flexible hamstrings and calves help to reduce falls by enabling for safer and more controlled movements when stepping over obstacles or getting up from a seated position.

5. *Facilitation of Recovery*

Flexibility also aids in the rehabilitation process following injuries or physical effort. Flexible muscles and joints are less prone to feel tight and uncomfortable after physical activity or injury. This freedom of movement can hasten rehabilitation and allow elders to resume their daily activities more quickly.

Example: Gentle stretching can alleviate muscle soreness and stiffness after physical activity, promoting a quicker return to daily routines and reducing the likelihood of prolonged discomfort.

6. *Enhanced Functional Independence*

Overall, enhanced flexibility promotes functional independence by allowing seniors to conduct daily activities more comfortably. Whether dressing, cooking, gardening, or participating in social events, seniors' flexibility ensures that they can move comfortably and efficiently.

Example: Flexibility in the hips and lower back can make it easier to bend down to pick up objects or get in and out of vehicles, thus supporting daily living tasks and maintaining autonomy.

7. Promotion of Mental Well-being

Flexibility exercises can also improve mental well-being. Stretching promotes relaxation and mindfulness, which can reduce stress and increase calm. This mental relaxation can supplement physical improvements by encouraging a more optimistic attitude on life and improving overall emotional health.

Example: Deep breathing combined with stretching practices can help you relax, reduce anxiety, and achieve a more balanced and happy mental state.

Identifying Personal Goals and Limitations

1. Assessing Current Fitness Level

Understanding Your Starting Point: Before setting goals, it's important to assess your current fitness level. This involves evaluating your flexibility, strength, balance, and overall physical health. You can do this through self-assessment, or for a more comprehensive evaluation, consider consulting a healthcare professional or a fitness trainer who specializes in working with seniors.

Example: Use a basic flexibility test, such as sitting and reaching for your toes, to gauge your current range of motion. Similarly, evaluate your balance by standing on one leg for a set period.

2. Setting Realistic and Achievable Goals

Short-Term Goals: Start with small, attainable goals that can be achieved within a few weeks or months. These goals should be specific and measurable, such as improving the range of motion in a particular joint or increasing the duration of a stretching routine.

Example: A short-term goal might be to increase flexibility in your hamstrings by a few inches or to stretch for 10 minutes daily.

Long-Term Goals: Set broader goals that focus on overall improvement over a longer period, such as six months to a year. These might include significant enhancements in balance, strength, or general physical fitness.

Example: A long-term goal could be to enhance overall flexibility and balance to reduce the risk of falls or to complete a 30-minute stretching and exercise routine consistently.

3. Identifying Personal Limitations

Physical Limitations: Be aware of any physical limitations or health conditions that might affect your ability to perform certain exercises or stretches. This includes joint pain, arthritis, muscle weakness, or any recent injuries. Understanding these limitations will help you avoid exercises that could exacerbate issues.

Example: If you have arthritis in your knees, high-impact activities or deep knee bends may be difficult. Choose low-impact stretches and exercises to meet your condition.

Medical Conditions: Consider any existing medical conditions that may affect your fitness routine. Conditions such as heart disease, osteoporosis, or diabetes can influence the types of exercises that are safe and beneficial.

Example: If you have osteoporosis, focus on exercises that promote bone health without putting excessive strain on the bones, such as gentle stretching and low-impact activities.

Physical and Emotional Energy Levels: Take into account your daily energy levels and overall well-being. Some days might be better suited for more intense activities, while others may require a gentler approach.

Example: On days when you feel particularly fatigued, it's okay to modify your routine to include lighter stretches or shorter exercise sessions.

4. Creating a Personalized Plan

Tailoring Your Routine: Based on your goals and limitations, create a personalized stretching and exercise plan. This plan should include a variety of exercises that address different aspects of physical health, such as flexibility, strength, and balance, while accommodating any limitations.

Example: If your goal is to improve flexibility and balance, your plan might include gentle stretching exercises, balance drills, and light resistance training, with modifications as needed for any specific limitations.

Incorporating Modifications: Adapt exercises and stretches to fit your individual needs. Use props such as chairs, straps, or stability balls to make exercises more accessible and to provide additional support if necessary.

Example: Use a chair for support during balance exercises or modify stretches to a seated position if standing is challenging.

5. Monitoring Progress and Adjusting Goals

Tracking Improvement: Regularly monitor your progress towards your goals. Keep a journal of your exercises, noting improvements in flexibility, balance, and overall physical health. Tracking progress helps you stay motivated and make necessary adjustments to your routine.

Example: Record your stretching times, range of motion improvements, and any changes in balance or strength over time.

Adjusting Goals: As you make progress, reassess your goals and adjust them as needed. It's important to remain flexible with your objectives and modify them based on your evolving fitness level and any changes in your health status.

Example: If you achieve a goal early, set a new one that builds on your progress, such as increasing the difficulty of stretches or adding new exercises to your routine.

6. Seeking Support and Guidance

Professional Advice: Consider seeking advice from healthcare professionals, such as physical therapists or fitness trainers who specialize in senior fitness. They can provide personalized recommendations, ensure that your routine is safe, and help you overcome specific limitations.

Example: A physical therapist can design a customized stretching program that takes your medical history and limitations into account.

Social and Community Support: Engage with support groups or fitness classes designed for seniors. These groups can offer encouragement, share experiences, and provide motivation.

Example: Join a local senior fitness class that focuses on stretching and balance to stay motivated and connected with others who share similar goals.

CHAPTER 3: SAFETY FIRST – PREPARING FOR YOUR STRETCHING ROUTINE

Warm-Up Essentials: Pre-Stretch Tips

To guarantee a safe and successful stretch session, adequately prepare your body before beginning. A well-executed warm-up helps to prevent injuries, improves the effectiveness of stretching activities, and boosts overall performance. Warming up is especially important for seniors over 60 since it prepares their muscles and joints for increased exercise.

1. Start with Gentle Movement

Purpose: Gentle movement gradually increases your heart rate, warms up your muscles, and enhances blood flow to the muscles and joints. This helps to reduce stiffness and prepares your body for more intensive stretching.

What to Do: Begin with low-impact activities such as walking in place, marching, or gentle stepping. Aim for 5 to 10 minutes of continuous movement. You can also incorporate light movements like arm circles or shoulder rolls to engage the upper body.

Example: Walk around the room or in place while gently swinging your arms for 5 minutes. This will help elevate your heart rate and prepare your body for stretching.

2. Incorporate Dynamic Stretching

Purpose: Dynamic stretching involves controlled movements that take your muscles and joints through their full range of motion. This type of stretching helps activate muscles, improve flexibility, and enhance coordination, making it an ideal complement to your warm-up routine.

What to Do: Perform dynamic stretches that target major muscle groups. Examples include leg swings, arm swings, and torso twists. These movements should be done gently and within a comfortable range of motion.

Example: Stand next to a wall or chair for support and gently swing one leg forward and backward, gradually increasing the range of motion. Do this for 10-15 swings on each leg.

3. Focus on Joint Mobility

Purpose: As joints are often more prone to stiffness and discomfort in older adults, focusing on joint mobility during the warm-up is essential. Mobilizing the joints helps increase fluid movement and reduce the risk of injury during stretching.

What to Do: Perform joint-specific mobility exercises such as ankle circles, wrist circles, and shoulder shrugs. Move through these exercises slowly and gently, paying attention to any areas of stiffness or discomfort.

Example: Sit in a chair and extend one leg out in front of you. Rotate your ankle in a circular motion, first clockwise and then counterclockwise, for 10-15 seconds in each direction. Repeat with the other ankle.

4. Use Proper Breathing Techniques

Purpose: Proper breathing techniques help relax the body and improve oxygen flow to the muscles. This can enhance the effectiveness of the warm-up and make the stretching routine more comfortable.

What to Do: Practice deep, diaphragmatic breathing throughout your warm-up. Inhale deeply through your nose, allowing your abdomen to expand, and exhale slowly through your mouth. Focus on maintaining a steady, rhythmic breath.

Example: While performing gentle movements or dynamic stretches, take slow, deep breaths in and out. For instance, as you march in place, inhale deeply with each lift of the knee and exhale with each step down.

5. Gradually Increase Intensity

Purpose: Gradually increasing the intensity of your warm-up ensures that your body is properly prepared for the stretching routine. This helps to prevent sudden strain on your muscles and joints.

What to Do: Start with very gentle movements and gradually increase the intensity of your warm-up as your body starts to feel more prepared. Avoid jumping into high-intensity exercises right away.

Example: If you're doing a warm-up walk, start at a slow pace and gradually increase to a brisk walk. As you progress, incorporate more dynamic movements like gentle leg lifts or arm swings.

6. Pay Attention to Pain and Discomfort

Purpose: It's important to listen to your body and avoid pushing through any pain or significant discomfort during the warm-up. Discomfort might indicate that you need to modify your routine or adjust the intensity.

What to Do: If you experience sharp pain or significant discomfort during any part of the warm-up, stop and assess. Adjust the movements or consult a healthcare professional if necessary.

Example: If you feel a sharp pain in your shoulder while doing arm circles, reduce the range of motion or switch to a gentler movement like shoulder shrugs.

7. Hydrate Before You Begin

Purpose: Proper hydration is crucial for maintaining muscle function and preventing cramps or strains during exercise. Drinking water before starting your warm-up helps keep your body well-hydrated.

What to Do: Drink a glass of water about 30 minutes before beginning your stretching routine. Avoid excessive caffeine or alcohol, as these can contribute to dehydration.

Example: Keep a water bottle nearby and take small sips throughout your warm-up and stretching session to stay hydrated.

How to Pay Attention to Your Health to Avoid Injuries

1. Recognize and Interpret Pain

Understanding Pain Types: Not all pain is equal. It is critical to distinguish between discomfort caused by normal exercise and pain that indicates potential harm. Acute pain, such as acute or stabbing pain, can suggest a problem, although gradual discomfort or soreness may be a typical reaction to new workouts.

What to Do: Pay special attention to the nature and location of the pain. If you suffer sudden, acute discomfort, stop immediately and assess. Mild muscle soreness, which occurs a day or two after exercise, is typically normal and indicates that your muscles are adapting.

Example: If you feel a sharp pain in your knee while stretching, cease the stretch and consult a healthcare professional to ensure there's no underlying issue.

2. Monitor Your Fatigue Levels

Recognizing Fatigue: Fatigue can indicate that you're pushing yourself too hard. Understanding the distinction between normal tiredness and extreme fatigue is critical for preventing overuse injuries. If you frequently feel depleted or exhausted after exercise, it may be necessary to reduce the intensity or duration of your activities.

What to Do: Pay close attention to how you feel during and after exercise. If you constantly feel exhausted, consider lowering the intensity or providing more rest between sessions. Make sure you're receiving enough sleep and recovery time.

Example: If you find yourself feeling excessively fatigued after your routine, it may be helpful to reduce the length or intensity of your workouts and focus on getting more rest.

3. Evaluate Range of Motion and Flexibility

Assessing Flexibility: Limited range of motion or stiffness may suggest that you are overextending or have not adequately warmed up. Maintaining a comfortable range of motion might help you avoid strains and injuries.

What to Do: Before stretching or exercising, evaluate your flexibility and range of motion. If you experience stiffness or difficulties moving across a complete range, it may be time to change your routine or extend your warm-up period.

Example: If you struggle to reach your toes while stretching, you might need to focus on gentle flexibility exercises and use props to support your stretches until your range of motion improves.

4. Use Proper Technique and Form

Importance of Technique: Using good technique and form when exercising and stretching is critical for avoiding injuries. Incorrect form can put undue stress on muscles and joints, resulting in strains or injury.

What to Do: Learn and apply proper techniques for all workouts and stretches. Consider hiring a fitness professional who specializes in senior fitness to guarantee that you're doing your workouts appropriately and safely.

Example: When performing a leg stretch, ensure that you maintain proper alignment and avoid overextending. If you're unsure of the technique, seek guidance to ensure that you're not putting unnecessary strain on your muscles.

5. Pay Attention to Body Signals

Listening to Body Cues: Your body frequently sends tiny cues that indicate whether you should continue or cease an activity. These symptoms can include muscle tightness, soreness, or changes in how your body feels while exercising.

What to Do: Be aware of these indications and change your actions accordingly. If you experience any discomfort or odd sensations, alter or discontinue the activity and consider consulting a healthcare practitioner.

Example: If you experience an unusual tightness in your back while stretching, modify the stretch or take a break to avoid potential strain.

6. Incorporate Rest and Recovery

Importance of Recovery: Rest and rehabilitation are essential for avoiding injuries and allowing your body to heal and strengthen. Overtraining or inadequate rest can raise the risk of injury and reduce overall performance.

What to Do: Include rest days in your training plan and pay attention to your body's demand for recovery. Allow enough time for muscles to recover between sessions, and include activities that encourage relaxation and healing.

Example: If you've had an intense workout or stretch session, allow a day or two for your body to recover before engaging in similar activities again.

7. Adapt Exercises to Your Abilities

Modifying Exercises: Tailoring exercises and stretches to your individual abilities and limitations helps prevent injuries. Avoiding activities that feel too challenging or painful ensures that you're working within your capabilities.

What to Do: Modify exercises as needed to fit your current fitness level. Use support such as chairs or bands to assist with exercises if necessary, and choose modifications that accommodate any physical limitations you may have.

Example: If a certain stretch causes discomfort, adjust the intensity or use a prop to make the stretch more comfortable. For example, use a towel to support your foot during a hamstring stretch.

8. Stay Hydrated and Nourished

Importance of Hydration and Nutrition: Proper hydration and nutrition support muscle function and overall physical health. Dehydration and inadequate nutrition can contribute to muscle cramps and fatigue.

What to Do: Drink plenty of water throughout the day, especially before and after exercise. Ensure you're consuming a balanced diet that includes adequate protein, vitamins, and minerals to support muscle health and recovery.

Example: Drink a glass of water before starting your stretching routine and include foods rich in calcium and magnesium in your diet to support muscle function.

9. Consult Healthcare Professionals

Seeking Professional Advice: Talking with healthcare specialists can provide individualized advice and address any specific issues or limits. Regular check-ups and consultations help to ensure that your workout plan is both safe and effective.

What to Do: If you have any underlying health conditions or experience persistent discomfort, consult with your doctor or a physical therapist. They can offer tailored advice and adjustments to your routine based on your health status.

Example: If you have a history of joint issues or chronic pain, a physical therapist can help design a safe and effective stretching program that accommodates your needs.

Choosing the Right Equipment and Environment

1. Selecting Appropriate Equipment

Comfort and Safety: Choose equipment that is comfortable and easy to use, with a focus on safety features. Equipment should be stable, non-slip, and designed to accommodate your physical abilities and limitations.

Types of Equipment:

Exercise Mats: A high-quality, non-slip exercise mat provides cushioning and stability during stretching and floor exercises. Look for mats that are thick enough to offer comfort but not so thick that they create instability.

Example: Choose a mat that has a textured surface to prevent slipping and is thick enough (at least 0.5 inches) to cushion your knees and back.

Supportive Chairs: For seated stretches or exercises, use a sturdy chair with a firm seat and backrest. Chairs with armrests and non-slip feet offer additional stability.

Example: A kitchen or dining chair with a solid base and comfortable padding can be used for seated stretches and balance exercises.

Resistance Bands: Resistance bands are versatile tools that can aid in strength training and stretching. Choose bands with varying resistance levels to match your strength and flexibility.

Example: Start with a light resistance band and gradually increase the resistance as your strength improves.

Hand Weights: Light hand weights can enhance strength training exercises. Select weights that are manageable and appropriate for your current strength level.

Example: Begin with 1-3 pound weights and adjust as needed based on your strength and comfort.

Foam Rollers: Foam rollers can help with muscle relaxation and flexibility. Choose a roller with a moderate density to avoid excessive pressure on sensitive areas.

Example: A medium-density foam roller is often suitable for seniors, providing enough firmness to be effective without causing discomfort.

Considerations:

Ease of Use: Ensure that the equipment is easy to handle and operate. Avoid complex equipment that may require advanced coordination or strength.

Adjustability: Look for equipment that can be adjusted to fit different body sizes and fitness levels. Adjustable features allow for customization and enhance safety.

2. Creating a Safe and Comfortable Environment

Space and Accessibility: Choose a space that is spacious enough to move around comfortably and free of obstacles. The area should be well-lit and easily accessible to minimize the risk of tripping or falling.

Environment Tips:

Clear the Area: Ensure that the space is free of clutter, such as furniture or cords, that could pose a tripping hazard. Keep the floor clean and dry to prevent slipping.

Example: Before starting your routine, scan the area for any potential hazards, such as loose rugs or uneven flooring, and remove or secure them.

Adequate Lighting: Good lighting is essential for visibility and safety. Ensure that the area is well-lit to help you see your movements clearly and avoid accidents.

Example: Use bright, even lighting to illuminate the exercise area. Avoid working out in dimly lit rooms where it might be difficult to see and navigate.

Temperature and Ventilation: Maintain a comfortable temperature and ensure proper ventilation in the exercise area. A well-ventilated space prevents overheating and helps you stay comfortable during your routine.

Example: Keep the room at a moderate temperature and open a window or use a fan to ensure adequate airflow.

Non-Slip Flooring: Choose flooring that provides good traction to prevent slipping. If possible, use non-slip mats or rugs in the exercise area to enhance stability.

Example: Use an anti-slip rug or mat under your exercise mat to provide additional grip and prevent the mat from sliding during use.

Accessibility Features:

Grab Bars: Install grab bars or railings in the exercise area for additional support and balance. Grab bars provide stability and help prevent falls during exercises or transitions.

Example: Install grab bars near the area where you perform balance exercises or transitions between exercises.

Supportive Furniture: Use furniture or equipment that offers support and stability. For example, use a sturdy chair with armrests for seated exercises and stretching.

Example: A chair with armrests can provide additional support when performing seated stretches or transitioning between exercises.

3. Personalizing Your Equipment and Environment

Assess Your Needs: Consider your individual needs and preferences when choosing equipment and setting up your environment. Your choices should reflect your fitness level, any existing health conditions, and personal comfort.

Example: If you have arthritis or joint issues, opt for softer, more supportive equipment, and ensure that your environment minimizes stress on your joints.

Seek Professional Advice: If you're unsure about the best equipment or environment setup for your needs, consult with a fitness professional or occupational therapist who specializes in senior fitness.

Example: A fitness professional can provide personalized recommendations based on your physical condition and goals, helping you select the most suitable equipment and environment.

CHAPTER 4: GENTLE STRETCHES TO START YOUR DAY

Morning Stretches to Kickstart Your Day

1. Seated Cat-Cow Stretch

Purpose: This stretch helps to gently warm up the spine and relieve morning stiffness in the back and shoulders.

How to Do It:

- Sit on a firm chair, feet flat on the floor, hands resting on your knees.
- Inhale deeply and arch your back, raising your chest and chin to the ceiling (Cow pose).
- Exhale slowly and circle your back, nestling your chin toward your chest (Cat pose).
- Repeat the cycle for 5-10 breaths while moving slowly and gently.

Tips: Keep the chair steady and avoid overextending your back. Move within your comfortable range of motion.

2. Standing Side Stretch

Purpose: This stretch improves flexibility in the side muscles and helps to open up the ribcage, enhancing breathing.

How to Do It:

- Stand with your feet hip width apart and your arms at your sides.

- Inhale, then raise your right arm overhead.
- Relax and bend to the left, extending your right arm above your head to deepen the stretch.
- Hold for 15–30 seconds before returning to the beginning position.
- Repeat on the opposite side.

Tips: Keep your feet firmly planted and prevent tilting forward or back. Concentrate on stretching through the side of your torso.

3. Gentle Neck Stretch

Purpose: This stretch helps to release tension in the neck and improve mobility.

How to Do It:

- Position yourself in a straight posture.
- Slowly tilt your head to the right, bringing your ear near your shoulder.
- Use your right hand to gently press on your left temple, intensifying the stretch if desired.
- Hold for 15-30 seconds and then switch sides.

Tip: Don't tug on your head or neck. Stretch only to the extent where you feel comfortable, and breathe deeply throughout.

4. Seated Hamstring Stretch

Purpose: This stretch targets the hamstrings and lower back, helping to improve flexibility and reduce stiffness.

How to Do It:

- Sit on the edge of a chair, one leg raised in front of you, heel on the ground.
- Maintain a straight back and softly lean forward toward your extended leg.
- Hold the stretch for 15-30 seconds and then swap legs.

Tips: Maintain a straight back and avoid rounding the shoulders. Use a chair with a firm seat to maintain stability.

5. Gentle Seated Twist

Purpose: This stretch helps to increase spinal mobility and alleviate tension in the back and torso.

How to Do It:

- Sit in a chair, feet flat on the floor, hands resting on your knees.
- Inhale deeply and straighten your spine.
- Exhale and slowly twist your torso to the right, resting your left hand against the outside of your right leg for support.
- Hold for 15-30 seconds, then return to your starting position and repeat on the opposite side.

Tip: Keep your motions slow and controlled. Avoid straining the twist, and only go as far as you feel comfortable.

6. Ankle Circles

Purpose: This stretch helps to improve circulation and flexibility in the ankles, which is particularly useful for seniors who may experience stiffness in their lower legs.

How to Do It:

- Lay on a chair, feet straight on the floor.
- Lift a single foot slightly off the ground and rotate the ankle in a circular motion.
- Perform 10-15 circles in each direction, then transfer to the opposite ankle.

Tips: Do the circles slowly and gently. Concentrate on performing smooth, controlled movements.

7. Chest Opener Stretch

Purpose: This stretch helps to open up the chest and shoulders, which can alleviate tightness from sitting or sleeping.

How to Do It:

- Emerge shoulder-width apart, arms extended to the sides.
- Inhale deeply, then slowly bring your arms back, pushing both shoulder blades together.
- Hold the motion of stretching for 15-30 seconds, then relax and repeat as desired.

Tips: Keep your shoulders down and avoid arching your back too much. Move simply to a comfortable stretch.

Easy Stretches for Improved Circulation and Energy

1. Neck Rolls

Purpose: To improve blood flow to the brain and relieve tension in the neck and shoulders.

How to Do It:

- ❖ Either sit or stand in a straight position.
- ❖ Slowly lower your chin towards your chest.
- ❖ Spin your head in a clockwise direction, first from one shoulder to the back, then to the other.
- ❖ Make 3-5 circles in one direction and then flip ways.

Tip: Move slowly and avoid jerky movements. Keep your shoulders relaxed and breathe deeply.

2. Shoulder Shrugs

Purpose: To increase blood flow to the shoulder area and relieve tightness.

How to Do It:

- ❖ Hold or get with your arms at your sides.
- ❖ Breath and raise your shoulders towards your ears.
- ❖ Vent and bring your shoulders back down.
- ❖ Do 10-15 times, focusing on the entire range of motion.

Tip: Keep your movements smooth and controlled. Avoid rotating your shoulders too much forward or backward.

3. Seated Leg Lifts

Purpose: To enhance circulation in the legs and strengthen the lower body.

How to Do It:

- ❖ Sit in a chair, back upright and toes flat on the floor.
- ❖ Stretch one leg straight out in front of you and hold for several seconds.
- ❖ Drop the leg and then switch to the other leg.
- ❖ Continue 10–15 times for each leg.

Tips: Keep your movements consistent and controlled. Avoid locking your knees and only elevate your leg as high as you can comfortably.

4. Standing March

Purpose: To stimulate circulation and engage the leg muscles.

How to Do It:

- ❖ Stand with your feet hip-width apart and arms at your sides.
- ❖ Lift one knee towards your chest, then lower it back down and lift the other knee.
- ❖ Continue alternating knees in a marching motion for 30 seconds to 1 minute.

Tips: Maintain a steady pace and use your arms for added balance. If necessary, hold onto a chair or wall for support.

5. Wrist and Ankle Rotations

Purpose: To increase blood flow to the extremities and improve joint mobility.

How to Do It:

- ❖ Extend one arm in front of you and make small circles with your wrist.
- ❖ Perform 10-15 rotations in one direction, then switch directions.
- ❖ Continue with the other wrist.
- ❖ For ankles, sit or stand and rotate each ankle in small circles, 10-15 times in each direction.

Tips: Move gently and avoid any sudden movements. Perform the rotations slowly to ensure full range of motion.

6. Chest Opener Stretch

Purpose: To enhance circulation in the chest area and alleviate tightness from sitting.

How to Do It:

- ❖ Stand with your feet shoulder-width apart and arms extended out to the sides.
- ❖ Inhale deeply and gently pull your arms back, squeezing your shoulder blades together.
- ❖ Hold the stretch for 15-30 seconds, then relax.

Tips: Keep your shoulders down and avoid overextending your back. Breathe deeply and maintain a comfortable stretch.

7. Seated Forward Bend

Purpose: To increase blood flow to the lower back and legs, and promote overall relaxation.

How to Do It:

- ❖ Relax in a chair, legs level on the floor, knees bent.
- ❖ Gently pull back from the hips, reaching for the floor or your toes.
- ❖ Hold the stretch for 15 to 30 seconds before returning to the beginning position.

Tips: Keep your back straight and just bend as much as you feel comfortable. Use a chair with a firm seat to provide support.

8. Gentle Side Bends

Purpose: To improve circulation in the torso and stretch the side muscles.

How to Do It:

- ❖ Stand with your toes hip width apart and your arms at your sides.
- ❖ Take a deep breath then raise your right arm overhead.
- ❖ Breath and lean gently to the left, extending your right arm above your head.
- ❖ Hold for 15–30 seconds before returning to the beginning position.
- ❖ Repeat on the opposite side.

Tip: Move slowly and keep your feet planted. Only stretch to the point where you feel comfortable.

Step-by-Step Guide with Illustrations

1. Neck Rolls

Purpose: To relieve tension and improve blood flow in the neck.

Steps:

- Starting Position: Sit or stand with your back straight and shoulders relaxed.
- Chin to Chest: Gently lower your chin towards your chest.

- Roll Head: Slowly roll your head in a circular motion, moving from one shoulder to the back and then to the other shoulder.
- Repeat: Complete 3-5 circles in one direction, then switch directions.

Illustration Idea: Show a figure sitting or standing with arrows indicating the circular motion of the head.

2. Shoulder Shrugs

Purpose: To release tension and improve circulation in the shoulders.

Steps:

- Starting Position: Stand or sit with your arms at your sides.
- Lift Shoulders: Inhale and lift your shoulders up towards your ears.
- Lower Shoulders: Exhale and lower your shoulders back down.
- Repeat: Perform 10-15 repetitions.

Illustration Idea: Depict a figure with shoulders rising towards the ears and then lowering back down.

3. Seated Leg Lifts

Purpose: To improve circulation and strengthen the lower body.

Steps:

- Starting Position: Sit on a chair with your back straight and feet flat on the floor.
- Extend Leg: Extend one leg straight out in front of you, holding it for a few seconds.
- Lower Leg: Lower the leg back down and switch to the other leg.
- Repeat: Perform 10-15 lifts for each leg.

Illustration Idea: Show a figure sitting on a chair lifting one leg straight out and then alternating legs.

4. Standing March

Purpose: To stimulate circulation in the legs.

Steps:

- Starting Position: Stand with feet hip-width apart and arms at your sides.
- Lift Knees: Lift one knee towards your chest, then lower it back down and lift the other knee.
- Continue Marching: Alternate knees in a marching motion for 30 seconds to 1 minute.

Illustration Idea: Depict a figure marching in place with knees lifted high and arms swinging.

5. Wrist and Ankle Rotations

Purpose: To increase blood flow and flexibility in the wrists and ankles.

Steps:

- Wrist Rotations:
- Extend one arm in front of you.
- Make small circles with your wrist.
- Perform 10-15 rotations in each direction.
- Repeat with the other wrist.

Ankle Rotations:

- Sit or stand with feet flat.

- Lift one foot slightly off the ground and rotate your ankle in circles.
- Perform 10-15 rotations in each direction.
- Switch to the other ankle.

Illustration Idea: Show a figure performing wrist and ankle rotations with arrows indicating the circular motion.

6. Chest Opener Stretch

Purpose: To enhance circulation in the chest area and stretch the shoulders.

Steps:

- Starting Position: Stand with feet shoulder-width apart and arms extended out to the sides.
- Pull Arms Back: Inhale and gently pull your arms back, squeezing your shoulder blades together.
- Hold Stretch: Hold the stretch for 15-30 seconds.
- Relax: Return to the starting position.

Illustration Idea: Depict a figure with arms extended out and slightly pulled back, showing the chest and shoulder area opening up.

7. Seated Forward Bend

Purpose: To increase blood flow to the lower back and legs.

Steps:

- Starting Position: Sit on a chair with feet flat on the floor and knees bent.
- Lean Forward: Slowly lean forward from your hips, reaching towards the floor or your toes.

- Hold Stretch: Hold the stretch for 15-30 seconds.
- Return: Slowly come back to the starting position.

Illustration Idea: Show a figure sitting on a chair leaning forward with arms reaching towards the floor.

8. Gentle Side Bends

Purpose: To improve flexibility in the torso and stretch the side muscles.

Steps:

- Starting Position: Stand with feet hip-width apart and arms by your sides.
- Raise Arm: Inhale and raise your right arm overhead.
- Lean to Side: Exhale and gently lean to the left, reaching your right arm over your head.
- Hold Stretch: Hold for 15-30 seconds, then return to the starting position.
- Switch Sides: Repeat on the other side.

Illustration Idea: Depict a figure leaning sideways with one arm reaching over the head, and then repeating on the other side.

CHAPTER 5: TARGETING KEY AREAS: NECK, SHOULDERS, AND UPPER BACK

Relieving Tension in the Neck and Shoulders

1. Neck Stretches

Chin Tucks: Sit or stand tall. Slowly tuck your chin towards your chest without rounding your back. Hold for 5 seconds, then release. This helps in realigning the neck and reducing forward head posture.

Neck Side Bends: Gently tilt your head to one side, bringing your ear toward your shoulder. Hold for 10-15 seconds on each side, repeating 3 times. This stretch releases the muscles along the sides of the neck, improving mobility and reducing tightness.

2. Shoulder Stretches

Shoulder Rolls: Sit comfortably and roll your shoulders in circular motions, forward 10 times, then backward 10 times. This promotes blood circulation and eases stiffness in the upper back.

Cross-Arm Stretch: Extend one arm across your body at shoulder height. With your opposite hand, gently pull the arm towards your chest. Hold for 20 seconds on each side. This stretch targets the deltoid muscles and helps release shoulder tension.

3. Upper Back Stretches

Seated Cat-Cow Stretch: Sit upright in a chair. On an inhale, arch your back and lift your chest (Cow Pose), and on an exhale, round your back and tuck your chin (Cat Pose). Repeat 5-10 times to stretch the entire upper back, relieving tension and improving posture.

Wall Angels: Stand with your back against a wall, arms at a 90-degree angle. Slowly slide your arms up and down the wall, as if performing a snow angel. This stretch helps to open the chest and strengthen the upper back muscles, which supports better posture.

Stretches for a Healthier Upper Back

For seniors, maintaining upper back strength and flexibility is crucial. Stiffness can develop with age, causing discomfort and a reduction in mobility. Frequent stretching helps promote better posture, reduce stress, and improve general health. The following are some efficient stretches made especially for the upper back:

1. Seated Upper Back Stretch

How to Do It:

- ❖ Sit in a sturdy chair with your feet flat on the floor.
- ❖ Clasp your hands together in front of you, rounding your shoulders forward.
- ❖ Hold for 15-30 seconds while breathing deeply.

Benefits: This stretch helps to relieve tightness in the upper back and encourages better posture.

2. Cat-Cow Stretch

How to Do It:

- ❖ Start on your hands and knees in a tabletop position.
- ❖ Inhale as you arch your back (Cow position), lifting your head and tailbone.
- ❖ Exhale as you round your back (Cat position), tucking your chin and tailbone.
- ❖ Repeat for 5-10 cycles.

Benefits: This gentle movement promotes flexibility in the spine and helps reduce tension in the upper back.

3. Shoulder Blade Squeeze

How to Do It:

- ❖ Sit or stand comfortably with your arms at your sides.
- ❖ Gently squeeze your shoulder blades together, holding for 5 seconds.
- ❖ Release and repeat 5-10 times.

Benefits: This stretch strengthens the muscles between the shoulder blades, improving posture and reducing upper back discomfort.

4. Cross-Body Shoulder Stretch

How to Do It:

- ❖ Stand or sit up straight. Bring your right arm across your body at shoulder height.
- ❖ Use your left hand to gently pull your right arm closer to your chest.
- ❖ Hold for 15-30 seconds and switch sides.

Benefits: This stretch increases flexibility in the shoulders and upper back, helping to relieve tightness.

5. Wall Angels

How to Do It:

- ❖ Stand with your back against a wall, feet a few inches away.
- ❖ Press your lower back, shoulders, and head against the wall.
- ❖ Raise your arms to form a "W" shape, then slide them up the wall to form a "Y."
- ❖ Return to the starting position and repeat 5-10 times.

Benefits: This exercise enhances shoulder mobility and encourages better posture.

Important Tips

- Always warm up before stretching, such as by walking in place for a few minutes.
- Focus on your breathing; inhale deeply as you prepare to stretch and exhale as you hold the position.
- Listen to your body; if any stretch causes pain, stop immediately and consult a healthcare professional.

CHAPTER 6: CORE STRENGTH AND STABILITY

Why Core Strength is Crucial for Seniors

Although core strength is frequently associated with sports and fitness fanatics, seniors, particularly those over 60, should also prioritize it. Nearly all physical activities are built on a strong core, which promotes stability, balance, and general functional movement.

1. Improved Balance and Stability

As we age, our sense of balance can decline, increasing the risk of falls. A strong core stabilizes the pelvis and spine, helping maintain balance during daily activities, such as walking, climbing stairs, or standing. Improved balance can significantly reduce the risk of falls, which are a leading cause of injury in older adults.

2. Enhanced Posture

Core muscles play a vital role in supporting proper posture. Weak core muscles can lead to slouching and misalignment of the spine, which can cause discomfort and pain. By strengthening the core, seniors can improve their posture, reducing strain on the back and neck.

3. Increased Functional Strength

Everyday tasks—like lifting groceries, getting up from a chair, or bending down—require core strength. A strong core enables seniors to perform these activities with ease and reduces the risk of injury. This functional strength is essential for maintaining independence and quality of life.

4. Reduction of Back Pain

Many seniors experience back pain due to weakened core muscles. Strengthening the core can help support the spine, alleviate pressure on the back, and reduce discomfort. Regular core exercises can lead to significant improvements in back health and overall comfort.

5. Support for Healthy Aging

Core strength contributes to overall fitness, enhancing endurance and vitality. By maintaining a strong core, seniors can engage more actively in social and recreational activities, fostering mental and emotional well-being. This active lifestyle is crucial for healthy aging.

Tips for Building Core Strength Safely

- Start Slow: If you're new to core exercises, begin with gentle movements and gradually increase intensity.
- Focus on Form: Proper technique is essential to avoid injury. It's better to perform fewer repetitions correctly than to rush through the exercises.
- Incorporate Variety: Engage different core muscles by including a variety of exercises, such as seated marches, seated leg lifts, or gentle twists.
- Listen to Your Body: If an exercise causes pain, stop immediately and consult with a healthcare professional or physical therapist.

Simple Core Stretches to Improve Balance

Improving balance, avoiding falls, and maintaining mobility as we age all depend on having a strong core. Stability and coordination can be enhanced by stretching the core muscles, particularly those in the hips, lower back, and abdomen. These easy, secure, and efficient core stretches were created especially for seniors over 60. Depending on your comfort level and range of motion, you can perform these exercises standing, sitting, or on the floor.

1. Seated Forward Bend Stretch (Chair Stretch for Lower Back)

This stretch gently activates the lower back and hamstrings, helping with posture and core stability.

How to Do It:

- ❖ Sit at the edge of a sturdy chair, feet flat on the ground.
- ❖ Slowly bend forward from your hips, allowing your hands to slide down your legs.
- ❖ Stop when you feel a comfortable stretch in your lower back and hamstrings.
- ❖ Hold for 20–30 seconds, then slowly return to sitting upright.
- ❖ Repeat 3 times.

Tip: Keep your movements slow to prevent dizziness.

2. Knee-to-Chest Stretch (Lying Down)

This stretch gently stretches the lower back and engages the abdominal muscles to improve core strength.

How to Do It:

- ❖ Lie on your back with your knees bent and feet flat on the floor.
- ❖ Slowly bring one knee toward your chest, holding it with both hands.
- ❖ Hold the stretch for 20 seconds, then lower the leg.

❖ Repeat on the other leg, 3 times per side.

Tip: If lying down feels uncomfortable, you can do this on a bed.

3. Seated Pelvic Tilt (Gentle Core Activation)

This stretch activates the pelvic muscles and abdominal area, helping to improve core strength and balance.

How to Do It:

❖ Sit on a chair with your feet flat on the ground and hands on your thighs.
❖ Tighten your abdominal muscles and gently tilt your pelvis backward (as if rounding your lower back).
❖ Hold for 5 seconds, then tilt your pelvis forward (arching your lower back slightly).
❖ Repeat the sequence 8–10 times.

Tip: Breathe slowly and avoid sudden movements.

4. Standing Side Bend Stretch (Lateral Core Activation)

This stretch improves flexibility along the sides of the torso, which helps with overall stability.

How to Do It:

❖ Stand tall with your feet shoulder-width apart and hands resting on your hips.
❖ Slowly bend to one side, keeping the movement controlled and smooth.
❖ Hold for 10–15 seconds, then return to center.

❖ Repeat on the other side. Do 2–3 rounds.

Tip: Use a chair or wall for support if you feel unsteady.

5. Cat-Cow Stretch (For Spinal Flexibility)

This yoga-inspired stretch improves spinal mobility and strengthens the core muscles.

How to Do It:

❖ Get onto your hands and knees on a comfortable surface like a yoga mat.

❖ Inhale as you arch your back, lifting your chest and tailbone (Cow position).

❖ Exhale as you round your spine, tucking your chin and pelvis (Cat position).

❖ Move slowly between these two positions 8–10 times.

CHAPTER 7: LOWER BODY FLEXIBILITY: HIPS, KNEES, AND ANKLES

Stretches to Enhance Mobility in Hips and Knees

Walking, getting out of a chair, and mounting stairs can all become more challenging as we age due to the stiffness of our hips and knees. Mobility can be maintained, joint discomfort can be decreased, and flexibility can be increased with mild stretching exercises that target these areas.

1. Seated Hip Circles (For Hip Loosening)

This exercise helps gently warm up the hip joints, increasing range of motion.

How to Do It:

- ❖ Sit on the edge of a sturdy chair with your feet flat on the floor.
- ❖ Slowly lift one foot slightly off the ground and make small circles with your knee.
- ❖ Circle 5 times in one direction, then 5 times in the other.
- ❖ Switch legs and repeat.

Tip: Keep your movements slow and controlled to avoid straining your hip joints.

2. Butterfly Stretch (For Hip Flexors and Inner Thighs)

This stretch targets the hip flexors and inner thigh muscles, which are essential for smooth hip movement.

How to Do It:

- ❖ Sit on the floor or a soft surface with your knees bent and the soles of your feet pressed together.
- ❖ Hold your ankles and gently press your knees toward the floor using your elbows.
- ❖ Hold the stretch for 20–30 seconds, breathing deeply.
- ❖ Repeat 2–3 times.

Modification: If sitting on the floor is uncomfortable, sit on a folded towel or yoga block to elevate your hips slightly.

3. Standing Hamstring Stretch (Knee Mobility Support)

Flexible hamstrings reduce stress on the knees and improve movement efficiency.

How to Do It:

- ❖ Stand in front of a low surface, such as a step or sturdy stool.
- ❖ Place one foot on the surface, keeping your knee slightly bent.
- ❖ Lean forward gently from your hips until you feel a stretch in the back of your thigh.
- ❖ Hold for 20 seconds, then switch legs.
- ❖ Perform 2–3 rounds per side.

Tip: Avoid locking your knee to prevent strain.

4. Hip Flexor Stretch (For Front Hip Mobility)

Tight hip flexors can restrict movement and cause discomfort. This stretch helps loosen the front of the *hips*.

How to Do It:

- ❖ Stand in a split stance (one foot forward, one back), with your hands on your hips.
- ❖ Slowly bend your front knee and gently lower your back knee toward the floor.
- ❖ You should feel a stretch in the front of the hip on the back leg.
- ❖ Hold for 20 seconds, then switch sides.

Modification: If needed, hold onto a wall or chair for balance.

5. Heel Slide Stretch (For Knee Mobility)

This stretch improves knee range of motion by gently engaging the muscles around the joint.

How to Do It:

- ❖ Lie on your back with both legs extended.
- ❖ Slowly slide one heel along the floor toward your buttocks, bending your knee as far as is comfortable.
- ❖ Hold for 5 seconds, then slide your heel back to the starting position.
- ❖ Repeat 10 times on each leg.

Tip: Perform this stretch on a bed if the floor feels uncomfortable.

6. Seated Marching (Gentle Mobility for Knees and Hips)

This seated exercise keeps the knees and hips moving without placing too much stress on the joints.

How to Do It:

- ❖ Sit in a sturdy chair with your feet flat on the floor.

- ❖ Slowly lift one knee toward your chest as if marching in place.

- ❖ Lower the leg and repeat with the other side.

- ❖ Do 10 reps per leg, alternating sides.

Tip: Keep your back straight and avoid leaning back.

7. Figure-Four Stretch (For Outer Hips and Glutes)

This stretch targets the outer hips and gluteal muscles, which are essential for hip mobility and balance.

How to Do It:

- ❖ Sit in a chair and cross one ankle over the opposite knee, creating a "figure-four" shape.

- ❖ Gently press down on the raised knee to deepen the stretch.

- ❖ Hold for 20–30 seconds, then switch legs.

- ❖ Perform 2–3 rounds on each side.

Maintaining Ankle Flexibility and Stability

In order to walk comfortably, keep your balance, and avoid falls, your ankles are essential. Our stability may be impacted as we age due to a decline in ankle joint strength and flexibility. Ankle mobility can be increased and stiffness, instability, and injury can be avoided with regular stretching and mild strengthening activities. Here are a few efficient exercises for seniors to keep their ankles stable and flexible.

1. Ankle Circles (Improve Range of Motion)

This simple exercise keeps the ankle joint moving smoothly in all directions.

How to Do It:

- ❖ Sit in a chair with both feet flat on the floor.
- ❖ Lift one foot slightly off the ground and slowly rotate your ankle in a circular motion.
- ❖ Perform 10 circles in one direction, then switch to the opposite direction.
- ❖ Repeat with the other foot.

Tip: Keep the movement slow and controlled to avoid strain.

2. Heel and Toe Raises (Strengthen Ankles and Improve Balance)

This exercise strengthens the muscles around the ankle and enhances balance.

How to Do It:

- ❖ Stand behind a chair or near a wall for support.
- ❖ Slowly raise your heels off the ground, standing on your toes. Hold for 2–3 seconds.
- ❖ Lower your heels and then lift your toes, keeping your heels on the ground.
- ❖ Perform 8–10 repetitions.

Tip: Breathe steadily and hold onto the chair if needed for balance.

3. Seated Ankle Alphabet (Gentle Mobility Exercise)

This fun exercise works the ankle joint in multiple directions to improve mobility.

How to Do It:

- ❖ Sit comfortably in a chair with your feet off the ground.
- ❖ Use one foot to "write" the letters of the alphabet in the air, moving from the ankle.
- ❖ Switch to the other foot and repeat.

Tip: Focus on slow and smooth movements. If needed, rest between sets.

4. Towel Stretch (Increase Ankle Flexibility)

This stretch helps improve the range of motion in the ankle and reduces stiffness.

How to Do It:

- ❖ Sit on the floor or a bed with your legs extended.
- ❖ Loop a towel or resistance band around the ball of one foot.
- ❖ Gently pull the towel toward you, keeping your knee straight.
- ❖ Hold for 20–30 seconds, then switch feet.

Tip: Avoid pulling too hard—stretch to a comfortable limit.

5. Ankle Rocking (Enhance Dorsiflexion and Plantar Flexion)

This exercise helps improve the movement required for walking and standing.

How to Do It:

- ❖ Sit on a chair with both feet flat on the floor.
- ❖ Slowly rock your feet, lifting your heels and shifting your weight to your toes.
- ❖ Then, lower your heels and lift your toes off the floor.

❖ Repeat 10 times in a slow, steady rhythm.

6. Single-Leg Stance (Boost Ankle Stability and Balance)

This exercise improves stability by strengthening the muscles around the ankle and foot.

How to Do It:

❖ Stand near a wall or chair for support.
❖ Lift one foot off the ground and balance on the other leg.
❖ Hold for 10–20 seconds, then switch legs.
❖ Repeat 2–3 times per side.

Modification: If needed, hold the wall lightly for balance or perform with both feet close together before advancing to one leg.

7. Resistance Band Ankle Press (Strengthen Ankle Muscles)

Using a resistance band helps build strength in the ankle joint, making it more stable.

How to Do It:

❖ Sit on the floor with one leg extended. Wrap a resistance band around the ball of your foot, holding the ends with your hands.
❖ Press your foot forward, stretching the band, as if pointing your toes.
❖ Slowly return to the starting position.
❖ Do 8–10 repetitions on each side.

Tip: Keep the movement slow and controlled to engage the muscles properly.

CONCLUSION

Being flexible and active as we age are crucial aspects of leading a healthy life. Stretching activities enhance balance, coordination, and general quality of life in addition to reducing stiffness and increasing joint mobility. These advantages are especially important for seniors over 60 since they promote independence, reduce the risk of falls, and make daily chores more pleasurable. whether for the hips, knees, ankles, or core, the stretches described in this book are made to be safe, efficient, and flexible enough to accommodate different skill levels. Even for a short period of time each day, incorporating these routines into your weekly calendar can result in observable improvements in range of motion, posture, and muscle relaxation.

But it's important to keep in mind that consistency is crucial. Stretching is a lifelong practice that changes with you rather than a one-time fix. Pay attention to your body, go at your own speed, and take pleasure in the minor accomplishments along the way, like walking a bit further, standing up straighter, or feeling more balanced. Before beginning a new exercise regimen, always get advice from your healthcare professional if you have any medical concerns or are new to exercising. Don't be afraid to utilize props like chairs, towels, or walls for support, and modify the stretches to fit your needs.

You can develop a stronger bond with your body, lessen stiffness and aches, and feel more confident and invigorated by including these easy motions into your everyday routine. How you take care of your body now and in the future is more important than your age. in order to improve your flexibility, mobility, and general well-being, take your time, stretch intentionally, and enjoy the process. One stretch at a time, here's to a healthier, more active future.

9 7983449 87934